Second Edition

and The London
School of Medicine and Dentistry

Anthony D Woolf BSc FRCP

Consultant Rheumatologist

Royal Cornwall Hospital

Truro, Cornwall, UK

MARTIN DUNITZ

© 1994, 2002, Martin Dunitz Ltd, a member of the Taylor & Francis group

First published in the United Kingdom in 1994 by Martin Dunitz Ltd, The Livery House, 7–9 Pratt Street, London NW1 0AE

Tel.:   +44 (0) 20 7482 2202
Fax.:   +44 (0) 20 7267 0159
E-mail: info@dunitz.co.uk
Website: http://www.dunitz.co.uk

Second edition 2002

A CIP record for this book is available from the British Library.

ISBN 1-85317-678-8

Distributed in the USA by
Fulfilment Center,
Taylor & Francis, 7625 Empire Drive
Florence, KY 41042, USA
Toll Free Tel.: +1 800 634 7064
E-mail: cserve@routledge_ny.com

Distributed in Canada by
Taylor & Francis
74 Rolark Drive, Scarborough, Ontario M1R 4G2, Canada
Toll Free Tel.: +1 877 226 2237
E-mail: tal_fran@istar.ca

Distributed in the rest of the world by
Thomson Publishing Services
Cheriton House, North Way, Andover, Hampshire SP10 5BE, UK
Tel.: +44 (0)1264 332424
E-mail: salesorder.tandf@thomsonpublishingservices.co.uk

Cover image: Artist's interpretation of an osteoclast attacking osseous tissue.

Printed and bound in Italy by Printer Trento S.r.l.

Contents

Introduction

As people get older they break bones, resulting in pain, loss of independence and sometimes death. This is the presentation of osteoporosis.

It is not inevitable. It is preventable and treatable.

This book is a guide to osteoporosis and its management. The facts are presented not only for doctors, but are also intended to aid discussion with patients to help them actively participate in their own management.

What is osteoporosis?

Osteoporosis is structural failure of the skeleton with increased risk of fracture. There is low bone mass and microarchitectural deterioration of bone tissue, leading to increased bone fragility (Figures 1 and 2).

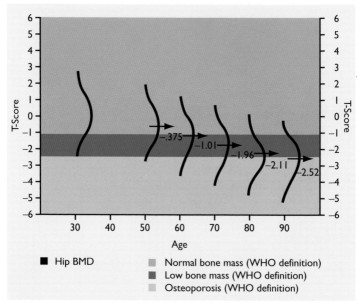

Figure 1 Bone mineral density changes with age, with WHO definitions of osteopenia and osteoporosis. Reproduced with permission from Osteoporos Int 1998; **8**(4)(Suppl.): S1–S88. © Springer-Verlag, 1998.

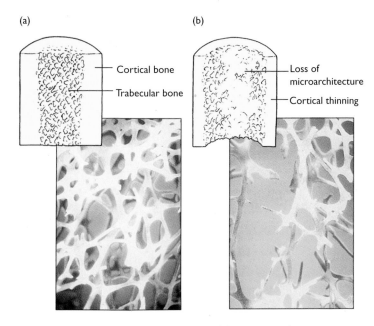

Figure 2 *(a) Normal bone in a 30-year-old; (b) osteoporotic bone in a 70-year-old.*

The World Health Organization (WHO) has defined *osteoporosis* as a bone density more than 2.5 standard deviations below the young normal mean. If an individual with a bone density below this threshold also has a fragility fracture, they have *established osteoporosis*. *Osteopenia* is defined as a bone mineral density more than 1 but less than 2.5 standard deviations below the young normal mean.

Osteoporosis presents as a fracture following minor trauma. The typical sites of fracture are the vertebrae, proximal femur and distal radius (Figure 3).

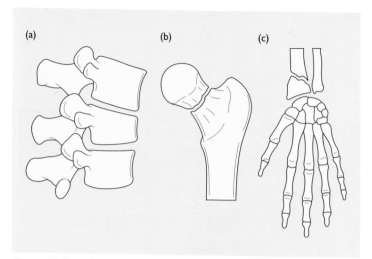

Figure 3 *Typical sites of osteoporotic fracture: (a) vertebrae; (b) proximal femur; (c) distal radius.*

Anyone over 50 years who has a fracture should be assessed for possible osteoporosis.

The size of the problem

Osteoporosis

Osteoporosis, a low bone mass, is the underlying cause of most fractures in anyone over 50 years.

The frequency of osteoporosis increases with age (Figure 1). The prevalence in British women aged 50–59 years using the WHO definition is 15%, rising to 70% in women aged over 80 years.

Fractures

Fractures are common, particularly among the young and the old (Figure 4).

Fractures among children and young adults are traumatic – usually sports injuries or road traffic accidents. Sites of fracture are the shafts of the long bones – mainly cortical bone.

Fractures in older people increase dramatically with advancing age. The 5-year risk of fracture in a 50-year-old woman is under 5%, but in a 75-year-old it is 15%. Women are more often affected than men. Sites of fracture are mainly trabecular bone – the ends of long bones and vertebrae. Osteoporosis is the major cause of these fractures (Figure 5).

Incidence rates for osteoporotic fracture differ between countries and races, but the age and sex differences are universal. In contemporary western society life expectancy has increased,

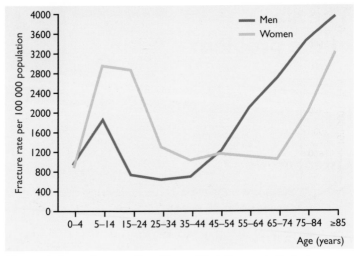

Figure 4 *Age- and sex-specific incidence of limb fractures in Rochester, Minnesota.*

with an increase in the elderly population at risk of osteoporotic fracture. Over the next 50 years it is projected that osteoporosis will become a major global burden with the rapid increase in ageing populations in Asia and Latin America.

The risk for a woman of an osteoporotic fracture is shown in Table 1 and is compared to that of other life-events; the risk for men is similarly shown in Table 2.

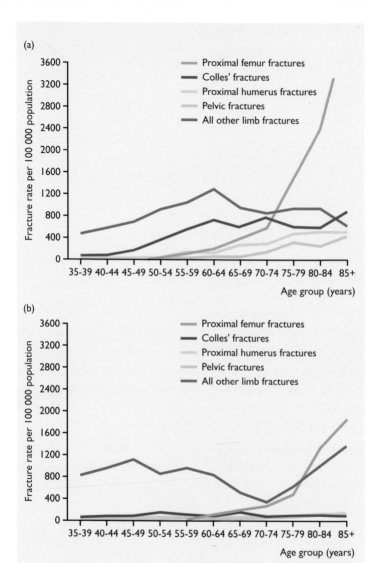

Figure 5 *Age- and sex-specific incidence of various age-related fractures in (a) women and (b) men.*

Table 1 *What is the risk for a woman?*

Event	Lifetime risk (%)	Cases per year (%)	Mortality (%)	Disability
Fracture of proximal femur	14	50 000	15–20 excess	+++
Colles' fracture	13	50 000		+
Vertebral fracture (clinical)	11	40 000	15–20	++
Any of above	35	140 000		
Breast cancer	8	16 000	40	+
Breast, uterine, cervical or ovarian cancer	15	24 000	50	+
Stroke	9			+++

Table 2 *What is the risk for a man?*

Event	Lifetime risk (%)	Cases per year (%)	Mortality (%)	Disability
Fracture of proximal femur	3	10 000	40	+++
Colles' fracture	2	40 000		+
Vertebral fracture (clinical)	2	8000		++
Any of above	10			
Prostate cancer	3			+
Stroke	12			+++

The development of osteoporosis

4

Osteoporosis (low bone mass and increased fragility) is a consequence of loss of the bone mass achieved by adulthood (peak bone mass).

Fracture occurs as a result of this bone fragility (that is, skeletal factors) and trauma (that is, extraskeletal factors), as shown in Figure 6 and Figure 12.

Osteopenia, or preclinical osteoporosis, is the term used to describe low bone mass and is defined by the WHO as a bone mineral density more than 1 standard deviation below the young normal mean, but less than 2.5 standard deviations below. Osteopenia is often used to describe what appears to be low bone density on an X-ray, but this is not a reliable way of determining bone density.

Osteoporosis is the term reserved for when the bone density is more than 2.5 standard deviations below the young normal mean. **Established osteoporosis** is often used to describe when a low-energy fracture has also occurred.

Skeletal factors

Increased fragility of bones results from:

- Low bone mass
- Changes in the quality of bone.

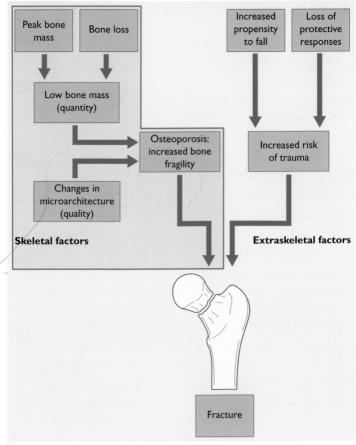

Figure 6 *Skeletal factors in osteoporotic fracture.*

Changes in bone mass with age

Bone mass increases during growth, consolidates over the next 15–20 years to reach its peak, and is then lost (Figure 7). As bone mass is lost, the risk of fracture increases (Figure 8).

Bone mass at any age is determined by the peak attained at midlife, the age of onset of bone loss and the rate of that subsequent loss. These are each influenced by different factors, as listed in Table 3.

Peak bone mass is determined by the genetic potential, but whether this is achieved depends on environmental factors such as mechanical stimulation, on diet, and on whether there are adequate sex hormone levels. There are several genes that influence bone mass.

The onset of bone loss occurs from the age of 40 onwards. There is a rapid period of bone loss in women following the menopause, and they have usually lost 30% of bone mass by the age of 70. Women have a lower bone mass than men at all ages, and fractures are more common in women.

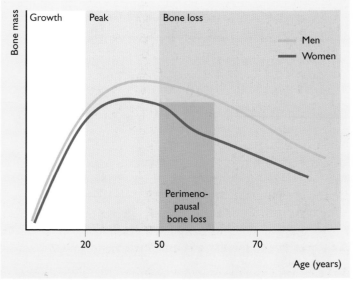

Figure 7 *Relation of bone mass to age in men and women.*

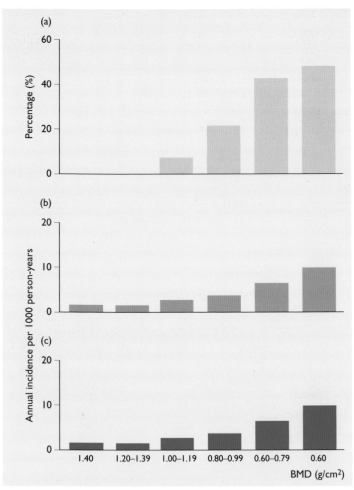

Figure 8 *The risk of fracture increases with lower bone mass in (a) the verte-brae, (b) the neck of femur and (c) the intertrochanteric femur.*

Changes in the quality of bone with age

Strength of bone depends not only on its quantity (mass) but also on its quality (microarchitecture), both of which deteriorate with age. Changes in the rate of turnover can affect bone quality.

Table 3 *Some of the factors that determine bone mass*

Peak bone mass
■ Genetic potential
■■ Candidate genes: vitamin D receptor, oestrogen receptor, collagen Iα1, PTH receptor, interleukins
■ Environmental factors determine attainment of potential
■■ Exercise
■■ Diet
■■ Sex hormones

Onset of bone loss
■ Age-related: men and women from 40 years
■ Menopause
■ Sporadic factors
■■ Immobilizing diseases
■■ Corticosteroid treatment

Rate of bone loss
■ Low levels of sex hormones
■ Immobilizing diseases
■ Reduced physical activity
■ Low dietary calcium
■ Corticosteroid treatment

The loss of microarchitecture has been illustrated in Figure 2.

With the loss of bone there is thinning and perforation of the trabeculae. The number of microfractures increases with age (Figure 9); if these microfractures fail to heal, the trabeculae lose their continuity (connectedness) and strength.

Bone is made of crystals of calcium and phosphorus – called hydroxyapatite crystals – embedded in a matrix of collagenous and non-collagenous proteins such as osteocalcin. Genetic

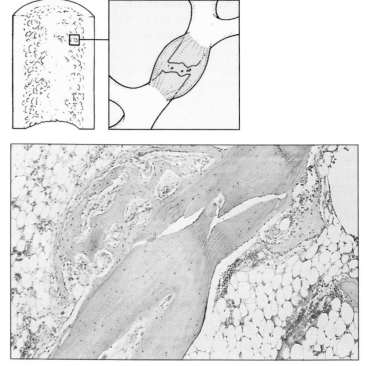

Figure 9 *Microfracture of trabeculae, with callus attempting to heal it.*

abnormalities of collagen also result in fragile bones (osteogenesis imperfecta). Furthermore, the collagen matrix of skin deteriorates with age, and this may also occur in bone and contribute to fragility.

Cortical versus trabecular bone loss

Bones are composed of an outer cortex of compact (cortical) bone and a rigid meshwork of trabecular bone (see Figure 2). These are found in different proportions throughout the skeleton. The shafts of long bones are mainly cortical bone. Vertebrae and the ends of long bones are mainly trabecular bone.

Trabecular bone is most active metabolically and is lost most rapidly at the menopause, with immobility and with cortico-steroid therapy. There is age-related loss of cortical bone from midlife onwards, with a slight increase in loss at the menopause. This differential loss of cortical and trabecular bone may result in the different ages at which fractures of the distal radius, verte-brae and proximal femur occur (Figure 10).

Mechanisms of bone loss

Bone is a living tissue that is constantly being renewed to main-tain its strength, and responding to mechanical stresses or injuries. It is also the body's calcium reservoir.

Old bone is removed and new bone is then made. This remodel-ling is performed by small groups of cells called bone remodel-ling units (BRUs) or bone multicellular units (BMUs). Initially, *osteoclasts* resorb bone and form a resorption cavity; *osteoblasts*

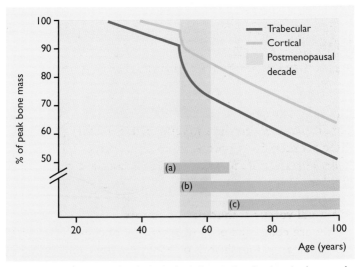

Figure 10 *The relationship between loss of cortical and trabecular bone and the ages at which different fractures occur in (a) the distal radius, (b) vertebrae and (c) proximal femur.*

are then attracted to the resorbed surface and synthesize bone matrix proteins and form a lattice or *osteoid* matrix; the newly formed osteoid then undergoes mineralization (calcification); the junction between osteoid and mineralized bone is called the 'calcification front' (Figure 11).

These processes of resorption and formation are normally closely coupled within these units so that there is no overall change in bone mass at the end of each 90–130-day cycle. The units are also asynchronous, so that at any time resorption at one site is normally balanced by formation at another, maintaining a constant total bone mass. This is controlled by many local and systemic growth factors.

For bone loss to occur formation and resorption are uncoupled, and either too much bone is resorbed or too little is made. How this occurs is not fully understood.

Osteoporosis may be caused when there is too little formation (e.g. due to ageing) or too much resorption (e.g. due to corticos-

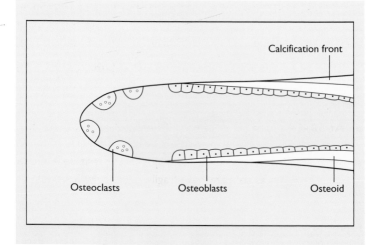

Figure 11 *Bone remodelling unit.*

teroid use or immobility). An increased number of remodelling units on the bone surface will lead to high bone turnover and loss, often combined with an imbalance of formation and resorption. This has important therapeutic implications, as some drugs stimulate formation while others impair resorption and reduce turnover.

Extraskeletal factors

Fracture is a result of trauma in addition to bone fragility (Figure 12).

The risk of falling increases with age. One in three elderly people will have a minor fall each year, most of them in the home, many of which result in fracture.

Specific causes of falls are occasionally found and should be looked for (Table 4), but most occur as a result of general musculoskeletal and sensory deterioration. Often more than one factor is involved, with an environmental cause being compounded with general deterioration or a specific medical problem.

The problem of falling is worsened by the loss of protective responses in the elderly owing to slow reflexes, poor orientation and loss of energy-absorbing soft tissues (fat and muscle).

What is the relative importance of these skeletal and extraskeletal factors in the causation of fractures of the proximal femur (Table 5)?

- **At 50–64 years** bone mineral density is the most important factor.
- **At over 75 years** falling is the major factor that determines who fractures, as so many have fragile osteoporotic bones.

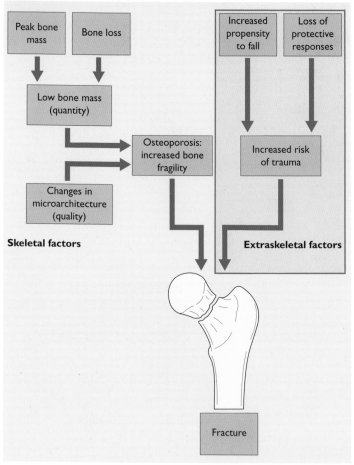

Figure 12 *Extraskeletal factors in osteoporotic fracture.*

Table 4 *Causes of falls in the elderly*

Intrinsic factors	
General deterioration associated with ageing	Poor postural control Defective proprioception Reduced walking speed Weakness of lower limbs Slow reaction time
Balance, gait or mobility problems	Joint disease Cerebrovascular disease Peripheral neuropathy Parkinson's disease Alcohol
Multiple drug therapy	Sedatives Hypotensive drugs Various comorbidities
Visual impairment	Impaired visual acuity Cataracts Glaucoma Retinal degeneration
Impaired cognition or depression	Alzheimer's disease Cerebrovascular disease
"Blackouts"	Hypoglycaemia Postural hypotension Cardiac arrhythmia TIA, acute onset cerebrovascular attack Epilepsy Drop attacks ?VBI

Extrinsic factors
Bad lighting Steep stairs Slippery floors Loose rugs Inappropriate footwear or clothing Tripping over pets, grandchildren's toys etc. Uneven pavements Bad weather Lack of safety equipment such as grab rails

Table 5 *Relative change in extraskeletal and skeletal factors that may contribute to fracture of the proximal femur, between 60–65 and 80–85 years*

Factor	Change (+/− %)
Risk of fracture of proximal femur	+ 1000
Extraskeletal factors	
risk of fall	+ 75
gait speed	− 35
strength	− 25
reaction time	− 20
Skeletal factors	
hip bone mineral density	− 30

Clinical aspects of osteoporosis

5

Osteoporosis presents as a fracture following a minor fall. It may be suspected by a plain radiograph showing increased radiolucency of bone (osteopenia, preclinical osteoporosis) before any fracture has occurred.

Osteoporosis does not cause symptoms, such as pain, unless a fracture has occurred.

Any fracture in a postmenopausal woman or elderly man should be considered as being due to osteoporosis and investigated and treated as such. At present, fractures following minor falls are not always recognized as being due to osteoporosis.

Common fractures are those of the proximal femur, distal radius, proximal humerus and vertebral bodies. Fractures of the proximal femur are associated with more deaths, disability and medical costs than all other osteoporotic fractures combined.

Causes of osteoporosis

The commonest cause of generalized osteoporosis is age, and it affects both men and women. Osteoporosis is more marked in elderly women as they have superimposed bone loss associated with the menopause.

Osteoporosis is idiopathic in the majority of women, but in up to 55% of men secondary causes are identified. The underlying causes of bone loss should be sought (Table 6), as they often manifest long before presentation with osteoporosis. Comorbidities that affect the outcome of osteoporosis and fracture should be identified. These are common in the more elderly and should be treated where present and possible.

Table 6 *Causes of generalized osteoporosis*

Cause	Example
Age	
Endocrine	Menopause
	Natural
	Surgical
	Radiotherapy
	Chemotherapy
	Primary and secondary hypogonadism
	Hypopituitarism
	Hyperparathyroidism
	Hyperthyroidism
	Cushing's syndrome
	Hyperprolactinaemia
Hereditary	Osteogenesis imperfecta
	Marfan's syndrome
	Ehlers–Danlos syndrome
	Homocystinuria
Drugs	Glucocorticosteroids
	Thyroxine in excess
	Heparin
	Alcohol in excess
Other	Myeloma
	Immobilization
	Anorexia nervosa
	Overexercise syndrome
	Rheumatoid arthritis
	Chronic obstructive airways disease
	Cystic fibrosis
	Post gastrectomy
	Coeliac disease
	Chronic liver disease
	Chronic renal failure
	Post transplantation
	Pregnancy

Bone loss may also be localized to a specific region of the skeleton without a generalized reduction in bone mass (Table 7).

Table 7 *Causes of localized osteoporosis*

Immobility/disuse*
Rheumatoid arthritis*
Algodystrophy
Transient regional osteoporosis
Pregnancy*

*Can also be associated with generalized bone loss.

Fractures of proximal femur

A fracture of the proximal femur presents as sudden pain with loss of mobility, usually following a fall. These fractures are very common, frequently disabling, and often associated with premature death (Table 8).

The incidence of these fractures is rising faster than the increasing number of elderly people in the population. There are approximately 50 000 fractures of the proximal femur each year in England and Wales, and with the increase in the numbers of the elderly alone it is estimated that there will be an enormous increase over the next 30 years, unless action is taken.

Table 8 *Fractures of the proximal femur*

Lifetime risk of women: 15%
Lifetime risk of men: 5%
90% occur in people aged 50 years and over
50% become disabled – unable to walk independently
20% lose independence
25–30% die within 6 months

These fractures not only cause morbidity and mortality but also consume large amounts of health care resources. The costs relate to acute hospital care and social support because of long-term disability and dependency. There are also hidden costs, as many orthopaedic beds are occupied by elderly persons following hip fracture, which prevents others benefiting from elective joint replacement surgery.

Fractured neck of femur represents less than 20% of total fractures in ageing women.

Fractures of distal radius (Colles' fracture)

A fracture of the distal radius usually results from a fall on to an outstretched hand. It is most common in winter, especially during icy weather.

The lifetime risk of suffering a Colles' fracture is approximately 15% for a woman, with a rapid increase in incidence at the menopause. It is the most common fracture in women under the age of 70: studies have shown that 20% of women have sustained a Colles' fracture by the time they are 70 years old.

Of these fractures, 20% result in hospitalization; most heal after 6–8 weeks, but some cause persistent pain and loss of function.

Vertebral osteoporosis

Vertebral osteoporosis does not cause symptoms until a fracture has occurred. In about a third of cases it presents as acute fracture with severe acute pain. In others it presents as progressive loss of vertebral height, with gradual loss of height, stoop, and often back pain. Vertebral fractures affect quality of life even if they do not present clinically.

The prevalence is 2–3% in women aged 55–60 years, rising to 20–25% in women aged 70, and affecting almost all women by the age of 80. Most will have also suffered fractures of the proximal femur or distal radius.

Acute vertebral fracture

Acute vertebral fracture (Figure 13) usually presents with sudden-onset severe back pain. It may follow minor trauma such as lifting or a sudden jar. The pain becomes worse with movement (including coughing or sneezing) and is eased by rest. Pain radiates with a dermatomal distribution (Table 9).

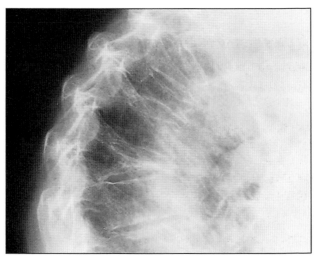

Figure 13 *An acute vertebral fracture.*

Table 9 *The dermatomal radiation of pain with acute vertebral fracture*

Area		Possible other cause
T5	Chest	?Myocardial infarct
T9	Rib margin	?Perforated ulcer
T11	Loin and umbilicus	?Acute abdomen
L1	Groin	?Renal
L3	Anterior thigh and knee	?Ureteric ?hernia

With acute vertebral fracture there may be associated shock, pallor and vomiting. There is usually spinal tenderness, with paraspinal muscle spasm and grossly restricted spinal movement. Neurological signs are absent and straight leg-raising is unaffected.

The acute pain usually begins to improve after 3–4 weeks and the fracture usually takes 3–4 months to heal.

Chronic vertebral osteoporosis

Chronic vertebral osteoporosis presents with loss of height and stoop (Figure 14).

There is often chronic back pain and all aspects of quality of life are affected. There may be chronic pain in the neck, which has to be hyperextended to look forward, or in the back. Loss of vertebral height results in compression of the abdominal cavity, and as a result there may be reflux oesophagitis, breathlessness, fullness with eating, and stress incontinence. The loss of space between the ribs and pelvic brim causes the abdomen to protrude, often with intertrigo in the skin folds and painful impingement of the ribs on the pelvis. The woman is usually distressed by her change in shape and apparently obese stomach. If she uses a corset, this will worsen the compression of the abdominal contents and the related symptoms.

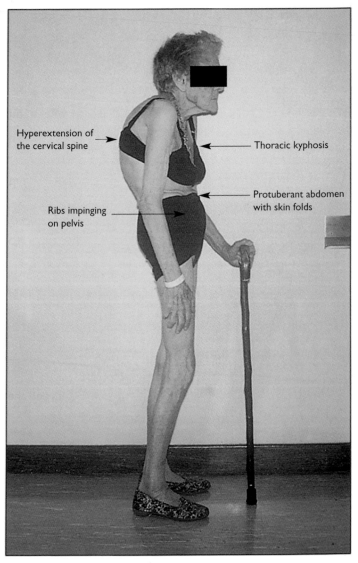

Hyperextension of the cervical spine

Thoracic kyphosis

Ribs impinging on pelvis

Protuberant abdomen with skin folds

Figure 14 *Chronic vertebral osteoporosis.*

Prevention of osteoporosis and fractures

6

All women, especially after the menopause, should take action to prevent osteoporosis, as it is so common. Men should also take action, as they have a significant risk of fracture. Osteoporosis is treatable but not reversible, and so primary prevention is most important.

Aims

The aims of prevention are to:

- Maximize bone mass and strength at all ages
- Prevent falls, maintain protective responses and reduce the impact of falls.

Maximize bone mass and strength at all ages

The maximization of bone mass should be undertaken at three stages (Figure 15):

- Maximize peak bone mass
- Delay onset of bone loss
- Slow rate of bone loss.

Peak bone mass

Peak bone mass is influenced by genetic potential, exercise, diet and sex hormones.

The genetic potential of an individual will determine the potential bone mass, but whether this is achieved depends on mechanical stimulation, on diet, and on whether sex hormone levels are adequate during growth.

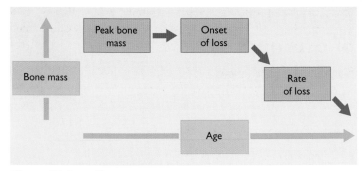

Figure 15 *Loss of bone mass.*

Exercise stimulates growth of the stressed bones (see page 53).

Calcium intake influences peak bone mass achieved (see page 72).

The reduction of exposure to female sex hormones (as in anorexia nervosa and gonadal dysgenesis) is associated with reduced bone mass, and the prolonged use of oral contraception is associated with increased bone mass. It is important to ensure that there are no prolonged periods of low premenopausal oestrogen levels. Sex hormones are similarly important in males.

Onset of bone loss
The menopause marks the onset of rapid bone loss in women. This can be delayed by hormone replacement therapy (HRT), with a reduction in the future risk of fracture, and replacement therapy should be considered by those at risk.

Rate of loss
The rate of bone loss may be slowed down at any stage by HRT, exercise or calcium supplements, and these are ways to prevent osteoporosis that should be considered by all women, especially if they are lacking in any of these. Bone loss is slowed down by bisphosphonates, SERMs (selective oestrogen receptor modula-

tors), calcitonin, testosterone or vitamin D (if deficient), and these can be considered to prevent fractures in those at high risk (see below).

Risk factors that may increase bone loss should be avoided: these include corticosteroids, excess alcohol, smoking, immobility and excess thyroxine.

In summary, one may recommend:

- Adequate exercise at all ages for both sexes
- Adequate calcium intake at all ages for both sexes
- Avoid premature deficiency of sex hormones
- Consider other treatments to maintain bone mass and prevent fracture in postmenopausal women at high risk of future fracture. These treatments are used for those with known osteoporosis or at high risk of osteoporosis, as they have been shown to be most effective in such people. Osteoporosis is best confirmed by measurement of bone density.

Prevent falls, maintain protective responses and reduce impact of falls in the elderly

The prevention of falls should be undertaken in five stages:

- Maintenance of fitness, balance and alertness
- Maintenance of vision and hearing
- Identify treatable causes
- Reduction of environmental hazards
- Reduce impact of falls.

Maintain fitness, balance and alertness

- Falls can be reduced by exercise programmes that concentrate on improving lower-limb strength and coordination. Exercises can also improve protective responses. A suitable exercise programme should be encouraged (for example, see pages 54–62).
- Consider walking aids and attend to feet
- Maximize mental stimulation

- Minimize sedation and other medication effects; advise on alcohol intake
- Check postural blood pressure
- Reduce bladder urgency.

Maintain vision and hearing
- Care with bifocal spectacles, as these often cause falls on stairs.

Identify treatable causes of falls
The likelihood of an elderly person falling is increased if he or she has already had a fall. It is therefore important to look for the causes of a fall and to try to prevent further falls in future from that or any other correctable cause.

There will be an identifiable treatable cause in 10% of cases, and an identifiable environmental cause in a further 10%. Most falls, however, relate to general ill health – more specifically, to sensory and musculoskeletal decline, with lower-limb weakness, unsteadiness and loss of protective mechanisms.

Causes must be looked for and treated to prevent further falls. A general examination should be carried out, including checks on pulse, postural blood pressure, vision and neuromuscular function. The drug history is important. A careful description of the fall from the patient or an eyewitness is an essential part of the assessment. Details of falls are correlated with possible causes and necessary investigations in Table 10.

Reduce surrounding hazards
This includes care with:

- Low obstacles
- Loose carpets
- Inadequate handholds
- Poor lighting
- Bath hazards
- Slippery floors.

Table 10 *Factors to investigate in a fall*

Detail of fall	Possible cause	Further investigation
Trip	Walking ability Vision Environmental	(see below) (see below) (see Table 4)
Loss of consciousness	Fit Stokes–Adams Hypoglycaemia	EEG ECG, 24-hour tape Blood glucose
Light-headed Faint	Postural hypotension Vasovagal Aortic stenosis Arrhythmia	Postural blood pressure? Drug history? Hypovolaemia? Addison's? Autonomic impairment? Preceding cough, micturition or pain? Followed exertion? Palpitations?
Palpitations	Arrhythmia Panic/anxiety	ECG, 24-hour tape Hyperventilation? Paraesthesia?
Head or body spinning (true vertigo)	Vertebrobasilar Insufficiency Vestibular disease Labyrinth disease	Related to neck movements? Related to posture? Nausea, tinnitus, hearing loss?
Legs gave way	Joint instability or pain Muscle weakness	Examine lower-limb joints Weakness, sensory deficit or abnormal reflexes? ? Spastic ? Neuropathy
Poor balance	Parkinsonism Cerebellar disease Cervical spondylitis/ Myelopathy Sensory neuropathy Gait dyspraxia (stroke, dementia)	Observe gait and transfers

Table 10 *cont*

Detail of fall	Possible cause	Further investigation
Poor vision	Cataracts Macular degeneration Wrong glasses Visual field loss	Check: acuity fields fundi tonometry

Reduce impact of falls

Hip protectors can prevent fracture of the hip and should be considered in recurrent fallers who have osteoporosis.

Who to target with preventive measures?

As osteoporosis is so common, all women (and also men at risk) should consider general measures that reduce the risk of fracture. However, not all women are affected and not all need or want to take HRT or other treatments, unless they are clearly at high risk. There are several treatments that will reduce the risk of fracture in those who already have a low bone mass or an osteoporotic fracture. Motivation to improve lifestyle and take preventive action is greater if the risk of osteoporosis is known. How can you identify those who will benefit most from treatment?

All established cases of osteoporosis who have already sustained a fracture should be assessed for osteoporosis and, if confirmed, treated to prevent further bone loss and reduce their high risk of further fractures (see Chapter 9).

All at most risk of future osteoporosis and fracture should be advised on preventive therapy. What is the best way to identify them before they have sustained a fracture or lost significant bone mass?

Low bone mass is the best predictor available of risk of fracture – for each decrease of 1 standard deviation in bone density there is a 2–3-fold increase in fracture risk. Other risk factors for fracture used either alone or in combination lack sensitivity and specificity, but can be useful to select those who should be assessed by bone densitometry. Some of them complement the use of bone densitometry. Risk of fracture is greatest in those with low bone density *and* clinical risk factors for osteoporosis, risk factors for falls or abnormal biochemical markers of bone turnover. It is generally agreed that population screening for osteoporosis is not appropriate but a number of risk factors (Table 11) can be used to help decide whether assessment by bone densitometry is indicated.

Bone densitometry is only indicated if the result will influence management. If a patient has already decided to take HRT because of a hysterectomy and oophorectomy at 45 years, then it is not appropriate. If strong risk factors are present, then a bone density result can allow an informed decision to be made. Compliance with treatment is increased following such informed

Table 11 *Clinical indications for bone densitometry*

Previous low trauma fracture over age 40
Osteopenia/vertebral deformity on X-ray
Loss of height, kyphosis if due to vertebral deformity
Glucocorticosteroid therapy (7.5 mg/day prednisolone for > 6 months)
Premature menopause (<45 years) not treated with HRT
Prolonged secondary amenorrhoea, such as anorexia nervosa
Primary hypogonadism (male and female) that has been untreated
Family history of osteoporosis, especially maternal hip fracture
Low body mass index
Disease associated with increased prevalence of osteoporosis (see Table 6, page 24)

decision making. Bone densitometry should be done only when an intervention can be recommended, and it is therefore inappropriate in premenopausal women unless there is a very specific indication, such as an eating disorder. Fracture prevention is more cost-effective if targeted in this way.

Bone densitometry

7

Bone mass

Bone strength and the risk of fracture relate to the mineral content of bone. Osteoporosis is defined by the WHO in terms of bone density. Bone density is the best available predictor of future fracture.

Bone densitometry

Bone density can be measured at different skeletal sites by a variety of methods.

Measurement at any site is most predictive of fracture at that site, but measurements at the spine, hip and forearm are predictive of fragility fractures in any part of the skeleton. The hip is the preferred site for diagnosing osteoporosis because of reproducibility of measurement and predictability of fracture. Measurements of the spine are affected in an ageing population by degenerative disc disease and previous fractures.

Bone mineral density (BMD) is measured as grams per cm^2, as it is only possible to measure the area of a bone, not its volume. Normal ranges have been established for different ages, genders and populations. BMD measurements are related to either young adults (T score) or age-matched individuals (Z score) of the same gender and expressed as standard deviations above or below the mean. Osteoporosis is defined by a T score below −2.5.

Indications for bone densitometry

Bone densitometry, like any test, is only indicated if it will influence clinical decision making.

There are several ways bone densitometry can be of use:

- To predict risk of fracture in individuals who have risk factors for osteoporosis
- To diagnose osteoporosis in an individual who has had a fragility fracture, vertebral deformity or osteopenia noted on an X-ray
- To monitor therapy.

A measurement of bone density is **predictive** of fracture risk for about 5 years, and repeating the test before then is of no value unless there has been a significant clinical change in risk. Bone-mass measurement does not fully discriminate between those who will and those who will not fracture, but the risk of fracture is more than 8 times higher in the lowest quartile than in the highest quartile. The indications are given in Table 11.

It is the only method to **diagnose** osteoporosis and identify the need for treatment with a bone-specific drug such as a bisphosphonate.

Monitoring of treatment can only be achieved by bone densitometry, improves compliance and is reassuring. The benefit of many treatments is, however, well established, and monitoring is not indicated in the management of uncomplicated cases. It is indicated for specific clinical reasons, such as unusual causes of osteoporosis, the use of novel treatments, or where it will influence clinical decision making. The ability of bone densitometry to demonstrate changes in bone density depends on the reproducibility of the technique and the expected change in bone density. For these reasons it should not be repeated in less than 18 months, and it may take 2–3 years to detect the effects of treatment.

Measurement of bone density

There are various ways to measure bone density, and dual-energy X-ray absorptiometry is the current method of choice.

Radiography

Plain radiographs are important in the diagnosis of established osteoporosis by demonstrating fractures, but they are insensitive for measuring bone mass, as 30% can be lost before it is noticeable.

Various methods to improve the sensitivity and reproducibility of radiography have been developed: these are metacarpal radiogrammetry, the trabecular pattern of the proximal femur (Singh index) and the measurement of vertebral body height. With the availability of dual-energy X-ray absorptiometry these are not now routinely used in clinical practice, although automated methods are being developed to improve the reproducibility of some of these methods.

Metacarpal radiogrammetry relies upon measurements of the cortical thickness of metacarpal bones, from which estimates of cortical bone mass can be made (Figure 16). This is simple and reproducible and there is an automated method.

The Singh index relies on the fact that there are characteristic changes in trabecular pattern as bone is lost from the proximal femur (Figure 17). This has been graded and related to the risk of fracture.

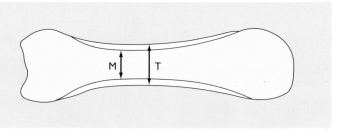

Figure 16 *The metacarpal radiogrammetry index. Total width (T) and medullary width (M) of second metacarpal are measured at the midpoint; the index is the ratio of M to T.*

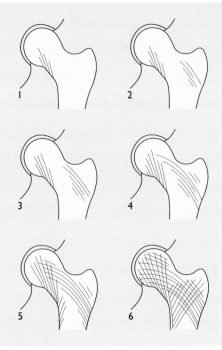

Figure 17 *The Singh index.*

Vertebral body height and shape can be used as an index of bone loss (Figure 18). A loss of more than 20% in height at the midpoint or anteriorly is defined as a fracture: some consider more than 15% to be abnormal. Various scoring systems have been developed for measuring loss of vertebral height. There are also automated methods of vertebral morphometry. Loss of vertebral height is called a *vertebral deformity*, as it cannot be certain when it occurred and it may be developmental and not represent a fracture, particularly in men.

Absorptiometry (densitometry)
The loss of radiation when an X-ray beam is passed through a bone gives a measure of the amount of bone mineral present.

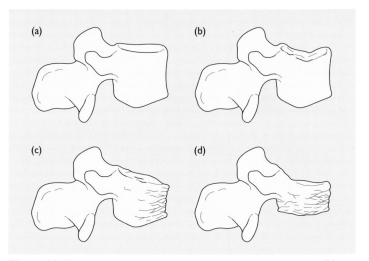

Figure 18 *Vertebral deformities as a result of osteoporosis: (a) normal, (b) endplate collapse, (c) a wedge fracture and (d) a crush fracture.*

Various methods have been used over the last few years. Dual-energy X-ray absorptiometry (DXA) (Figure 19) is fast and precise and is currently the recommended method. It involves little radiation and can measure bone density at any site. The proximal femur and lumbar spine are used, as they are the best predictors of fracture at those sites. Mobile machines can measure the distal forearm and calcaneus. The proximal femur is the site that is most reproducible and the best predictor of hip fracture – the most devastating of the osteoporotic fractures.

Quantitative computerized tomography (qCT)
Computerized tomography can be used to measure the vertebral bone mineral content and to assess cortical and trabecular bone separately. It is slow, and there is significant radiation if it is to be used for screening healthy people or for repeat measurements. Peripheral qCT will measure trabecular and cortical bone at the distal radius with low radiation.

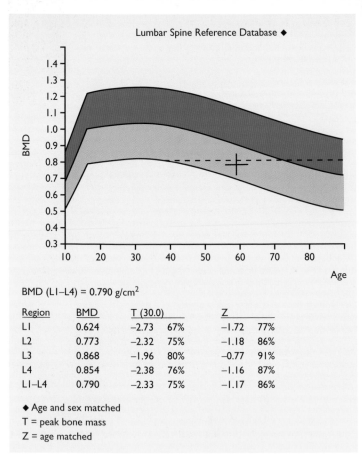

BMD (L1–L4) = 0.790 g/cm^2

Region	BMD	T (30.0)		Z	
L1	0.624	–2.73	67%	–1.72	77%
L2	0.773	–2.32	75%	–1.18	86%
L3	0.868	–1.96	80%	–0.77	91%
L4	0.854	–2.38	76%	–1.16	87%
L1–L4	0.790	–2.33	75%	–1.17	86%

◆ Age and sex matched
T = peak bone mass
Z = age matched

Figure 19 *Volumetric analysis of lumbar spinal bone mineral density by DXA.*

Ultrasound

Ultrasound is a simple method that measures the attenuation of ultrasound by bone: it can separate high and low bone mass and may estimate the risk of fracture. It cannot diagnose osteoporosis, as it is not measuring bone mineral content. There are a variety of machines that assess different skeletal sites: at present there is insufficient cross-calibration to be able to recommend any single site or method, but there are most data available for the calcaneus.

Management of established osteoporosis

8

Osteoporosis is a reduced bone mass with increased risk of fracture. It is not usually diagnosed until a fracture has occurred, and then it is called established osteoporosis. Any fracture in a postmenopausal woman or elderly man should be considered as being due to osteoporosis and managed as such. Although it is not reversible, much can be done to help the patient and to prevent the condition worsening. The risk of a further osteoporotic fracture is high.

The management of osteoporosis involves confirming the diagnosis, excluding other causes of back pain, stoop, bone pain, fracture or osteopenia, and looking for specific causes of osteoporosis. Treatment is to relieve symptoms and to reduce the risk of fracture (Figure 20).

Diagnosis of osteoporosis

In the investigation of the cause of bone or back pain, a fracture must be demonstrated on a plain radiograph for symptoms to be attributed to osteoporosis. Osteoporosis without fracture does not cause pain.

In the investigation for possible low bone mass (that is, someone with a predisposing condition (see Table 6) or osteopenia on radiograph), then bone mass measurement is needed to confirm osteoporosis. This is by bone densitometry (for further details see page 39).

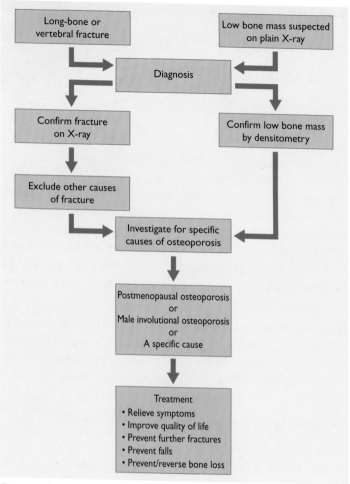

Figure 20 *Management of established osteoporosis.*

Radiographs may show an increased trabecular pattern in early osteoporosis, but 30% of bone mass can be lost before it is evident on a plain radiograph. Vertebrae may show endplate deformities, anterior wedging or crush fractures.

Table 12 *Differential diagnosis of fracture and vertebral deformity*

Osteoporosis
Primary malignancy including myeloma
Metastatic malignancy – breast, prostate, lung and renal most common
Osteomalacia
Paget's disease
Osteomyelitis
Traumatic vertebral fracture earlier in life
Scheuermann's osteochondritis of the spine

Radiographs will not indicate whether the fracture is recent, but an isotope bone scan will show increased uptake for several weeks after a fracture. Radiography may reveal lytic lesions, and a PA view of the spine may demonstrate pedicles that have been destroyed by metastases.

Other causes of fracture or vertebral deformity must be excluded (Table 12). This includes a full examination, in particular the breasts or prostate, and the appropriate haematology and biochemistry investigations (Table 13). In postmenopausal and age-related osteoporosis these should be normal (Table 14).

The cause of osteoporosis should be sought (Table 6, page 24).

Treatment of established osteoporosis

The aims of treatment are to relieve symptoms; in particular, to control pain, to improve quality of life by tackling functional and practical problems, and to prevent further fractures by preventing falls and the reversal of bone loss.

The methods of treatment are to assess the problems caused by osteoporosis, in particular pain and functional impairment. Treatment can be divided into:

Table 13 *Investigation of fracture or bone pain*

Investigations need to be tailored to the individual, depending on site of fracture and if other findings suggest a pathological cause

Baseline

- Full examination, in particular breasts or prostate
- X-ray of affected site
- Haematology
  - full blood count
  - viscosity or ESR
- Biochemistry
  - serum calcium, phosphate
  - serum alkaline phosphatase
  - serum creatinine
  - serum albumin
  - testosterone and SHBG in men

Further assessment

- Further imaging
  - Isotope bone scan – if any concern about metastases
  - CT scan or MRI to characterize lesion
- Biochemistry
  - liver function tests
  - serum protein electrophoresis
  - thyroid function tests
  - urine Bence-Jones protein
  - prostate-specific antigen (PSA) in men with vertebral fractures

Table 14 *Biochemical changes in bone disease*

Disease	Plasma calcium	Plasma phosphate	Plasma alkaline phosphatase	Viscosity or ESR	Other investigations
Osteoporosis	N	N	N	N	DXA
Osteomalacia	N or ↓	N or ↓	N or ↑	N	Serum vitamin D Bone biopsy
Paget's disease	N or ↑	N	↑	N	
Primary hyperparathyroidism	↑	N or ↓	N or ↑	N	Parathyroid hormone ↑ (PTH)
Myeloma	N or ↑	N or ↑	N or ↑	N or ↑	Serum protein electrophoresis Urine Bence-Jones protein
Malignancy	N or ↗	N	N or ↗	N or ↗	Breast examination Prostate-specific antigen (PSA) Chest X-ray Bone scintigraphy

ESR = erythrocyte sedimentation rate

49

- Explanation to and education of the patient and their partner or carer
- Adequate pain control
- Functional assessment and practical advice
- Physiotherapy advice and exercise regimens
- Prevention of falls
- Prevention and attempted reversal of bone loss.

Adequate treatment should be given to inhibit (or slow down) the progression of the disease and to reduce the risk of fractures.

Patient education

A patient can cope much better with a chronic painful disabling disease if they have a good understanding of it. Certain questions frequently arise and it may be helpful to have some brief answers available.

What is osteoporosis?

Thinning and weakness of bones.

What problems does it cause?

Broken bones
Loss of height and stoop

- with back or neck pain
- with protuberant abdomen
- with reflux oesophagitis
- with stress incontinence.

Can it be treated?

Yes, but it cannot be reversed
The problems it causes can be treated
Further loss and weakening of the bones can be slowed
Risk of future fracture can be reduced at any age.

What will happen to me, will I lose independence?

There is a risk of further fracture but this will not necessarily happen: there are effective treatments to prevent fracture and ways of helping people stay independent:

- Explain that it is not the same as osteoarthritis or disc degeneration – a common misunderstanding.
- Take a positive approach to the person with osteoporosis.
- A better understanding of the problem helps not only the individual with osteoporosis but also the carer to cope with something that is not curable.

See further questions and answers on pages 79–81.

Pain control

Patients and doctors often underestimate the suffering that chronic pain causes. Patients tend to avoid analgesics if they are told to take them 'only when the pain is bad' and hence under-treat their pain. Ask patients to score minimum and maximum pain separately on a scale of 0 (none) to 10 (worst pain ever): this helps them to put their pain into a proper perspective and to control it appropriately.

Analgesics should be selected according to the severity of pain and the response to previous treatment. The spectrum is: simple analgesics, NSAIDs, opiates (often necessary for an acute fracture), nerve blocks or transcutaneous nerve stimulation (TNS). NSAIDs with a low or minimal risk of gastrointestinal side-effects, such as COX-2 selective NSAIDs, should be used in this age group.

Acute vertebral fracture often requires bed rest and opiates for the first few days. Calcitonin (100 IU daily by injection for 3 weeks) has some analgesic effects. Adequate analgesia should be used to enable rapid restoration of mobility.

Physiotherapy – heat, ultrasound and massage – will help to reduce muscle spasm.

Corsets seldom help.

Local nerve blocks may help pain control following vertebral fracture. Tricyclic antidepressants (amitriptyline 25–75 mg nocte, dothiepin 75–150 mg nocte) may improve pain control, but always ensure they do not cause daytime sedation with increased risk of falling.

Functional and practical problems and advice

It is important to assess and discuss the problems of everyday life. Many lose independence following fracture, especially a fractured neck of femur. They will need intensive rehabilitation immediately after the surgical recovery period, and may require home assessment if independence is to be maintained.

Many activities become difficult following vertebral fracture. The following are some simple suggestions.

Clothing Advise patients to wear loose-fitting clothes. Corsets should be avoided, as they compress the protuberant abdomen and support the lumbar spine, whereas it is the thoracic spine that is usually most affected by osteoporotic vertebral collapse.

Seating Seating should be of the correct height, be firm, and give good support to the back, thighs and head.

Standing Advise patients to use perching stools, shooting sticks and public seating if prolonged standing is a problem.

Cooking It is best to avoid high cupboards and to use working-level appliances, microwaves and lightweight cooking pans. A lower work surface may be easier.

Cleaning Advise patients to use a long-handled brush and dustpan.

Bathing Advise patients to use a shower or a bath seat. A long-handled brush, flannel or sponge can help.

Sleeping This may be helped by a firm but not too hard mattress, a lightweight duvet and a neck pillow.

Walking It is important to avoid falling or any sudden jars. Walking sticks encourage an upright posture if they are of the correct height, and they give confidence and stability.

Carrying Advise patients to avoid heavy loads; to lift using their knees and not their back; and to avoid stooping.

Appliances A collar or a neck pillow used at night will help relieve neck pain. A collar may also sometimes be helpful in the daytime.

Refer patients to an occupational therapist if there is significant functional limitation.

Further advice to sufferers is available in most countries through their national osteoporosis organizations, the details of which can be obtained from the International Osteoporosis Foundation (see page 81). In the United Kingdom a wide range of booklets and a telephone helpline are provided by the National Osteoporosis Society (see page 81).

Physiotherapy advice and exercise in osteoporosis
The aim of physiotherapy is to reduce symptoms and disability, and increasing physical activity reduces bone loss and the risk of falling. There is often fear of exercise because of pain, or it may be restricted by other problems such as arthritis or angina, and advice from a physiotherapist can help establish an appropriate exercise programme. Hydrotherapy is especially suitable if the patient is in pain and mobility is restricted.

General exercise should be encouraged, and a programme can be found in many sources. The important points are that it should be weight-bearing and performed for at least 30 minutes per day. One of the simplest exercises is hard walking. Group exercise has benefits of motivation and social contact, with greater compliance: it can be done in a hospital or community centre, with supervision by a suitably qualified instructor. Any exercise must not increase the risk of falling or put excessive stress on to any one bone.

Specific exercises for vertebral osteoporosis should also be encouraged. The important points that should be included in any exercise programme are:

- Relaxation to relieve muscle spasm
- Monitor height and posture
- Breathing exercises
- Strengthening of postural (legs, back and abdominals), pelvic floor, shoulder girdle and neck muscles
- Avoid manipulation – the vertebrae are fragile!

Exercise regimen for vertebral osteoporosis

The following is a suggested exercise programme for vertebral osteoporosis, to be performed daily. The exercises should be tried cautiously at first, preferably under supervision, and then performed regularly if they do not aggravate symptoms and are not too exhausting.

Posture

It is important to monitor height and posture.

Exercise Stand with your back against the wall and try to make your heels, bottom, shoulders and head touch the wall at the same time (Figure 21). Walk forwards and then backwards to the wall to see if you can keep that upright posture.

The postural muscles are the legs, back and abdominals, and these may be strengthened by other exercises.

Standing

Standing exercises strengthen muscles in the legs, back and arms.

Exercise Swing your arms above your head, stretch and lower them; breathe in as you lift, breathe out as you lower (Figure 22a).

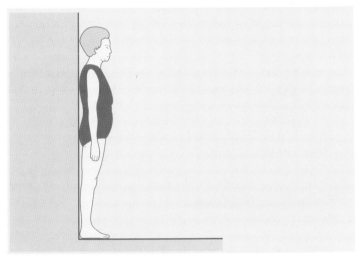

Figure 21 *(postural exercise)*

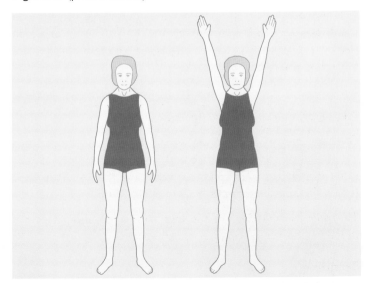

Figure 22a *(standing exercises)*

Side-bends to alternate sides; keep your heels down and stretch your hand towards your knee (Figure 22b).

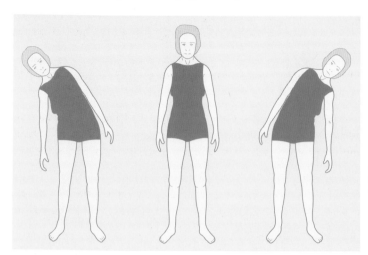

Figure 22b

March on the spot to a count of 30 and lift your feet as high as you can; hold on to the back of a chair if you need to steady yourself (Figure 22c).

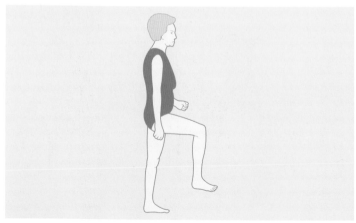

Figure 22c

Sitting

Sitting exercises strengthen the arms, neck and shoulder girdle.

Exercise Hands on your waist: slump forward and down; sit up straight and arch backwards; shoulders back and look upwards (Figure 23a).

Hands on your waist: twist round to the right, then to the left (Figure 23b).

Hands on the bottom of your ribcage: breathe in through your nose; feel your ribs expand outwards; breathe out through your mouth: gently squeeze inwards with your hand to help press the air out (Figure 23c).

Straighten one leg out in front of you, pulling your toes up towards you while bracing your knee; gently let your knee bend and repeat with the other leg (Figure 23d).

Sitting up straight, hands on your thighs: tip your head backwards gently; then tip your chin forwards and down (Figure 23e).

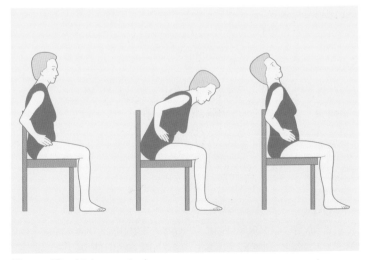

Figure 23a *(sitting exercises)*

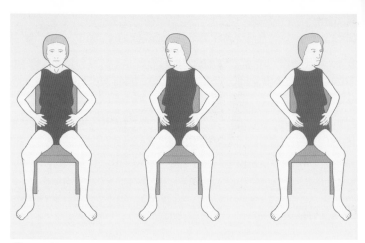

Figure 23b

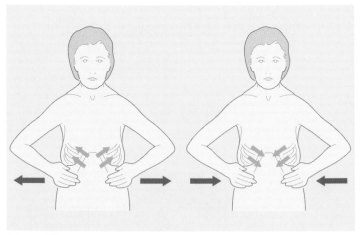

Figure 23c

Sitting up straight: push your chin forwards; then press your head backwards (so that you feel a stretch at the back of your neck); give yourself a double chin (Figure 23f)!!

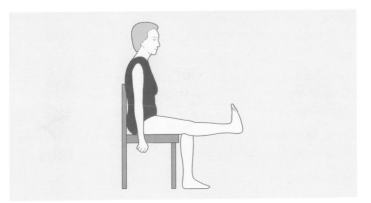

Figure 23d

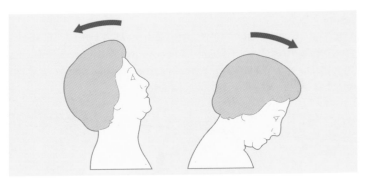

Figure 23e

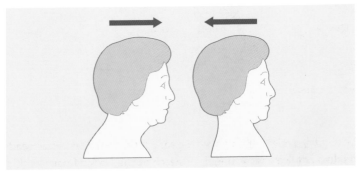

Figure 23f

Lying

Lying exercises strengthen the legs, back and abdominal muscles.

Exercise Knees bent, feet flat: arch the small of your back away from the floor, then press it down into the floor; tighten your stomach muscles as this will help you to press down harder (Figure 24a).

Knees bent, feet flat: lift your bottom off the floor as high as you can and arch your back; hold and then lower (Figure 24b).

Knees bent, feet flat: roll both knees from side to side; keep your knees and feet together (Figure 24c).

Legs out straight: brace your knees down into the floor, pulling your toes up towards you; hold and then release (Figure 24d).

Legs out straight, hands on your thighs: stretch both arms above your head; stretch your fingers and toes away from you; hold and then relax and lower your arms; breathe in as you lift your arms and out as you lower them (Figure 24e).

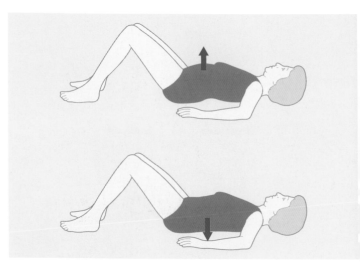

Figure 24a *(lying exercises)*

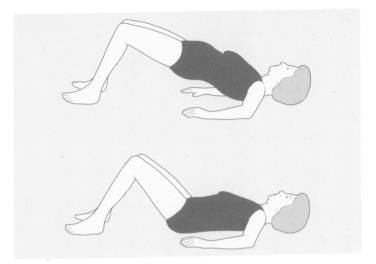

Figure 24b

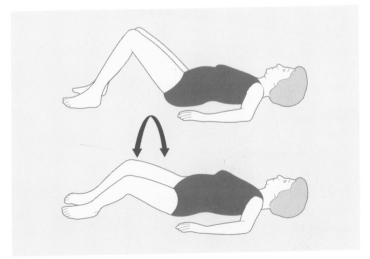

Figure 24c

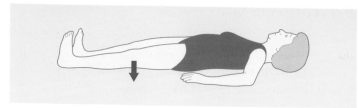

Figure 24d

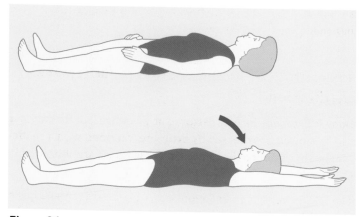

Figure 24e

Pelvic floor

Pelvic floor exercises strengthen the muscles and reduce the risk of stress incontinence.

Exercise Tighten the muscles between your legs as though you are stopping yourself from going to the toilet, then clench the cheeks of your bottom together, hold for 5 seconds and then relax and repeat.

Prevention of falls

The likelihood of an elderly person falling is increased if he or she has fallen already. It is therefore important to look for the causes of a fall and to try to prevent further falls in the future from that or any other correctable cause (see page 33).

Falls can be reduced by exercise programmes that concentrate on improving lower limb strength and coordination.

The impact of falls can be reduced by hip protectors, and these should be considered in someone who is a recurrent faller and has underlying osteoporosis.

Prevention of further bone loss/adequate medication

Bone loss cannot be fully restored at this stage, but further loss can be slowed or reversed by drug interventions, with a reduction in the risk of further fracture. These issues are discussed in Chapter 9.

The minimum recommendation is that the patient should begin weight-bearing exercise (see page 53), maintain a calcium intake of at least 1 g daily, and ensure adequate dietary vitamin D (800 IU in the frail elderly).

If the patient has had a hysterectomy, continuous oestrogens should be considered.

If the patient has not had a hysterectomy, one should consider other treatments such as continuous combination hormone replacement therapy (HRT), livial, raloxifene, bisphosphonates (including etidronate, alendronate and risedronate), calcitonin, and testosterone if male.

These treatments should, if possible, be initiated after the diagnosis of osteoporosis has been confirmed and other causes of fracture excluded (see page 47).

Treatments

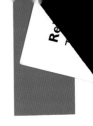

Hormone replacement therapy

Bone loss increases at the menopause, and is most marked following a surgically induced menopause. Bone loss is prevented by HRT, and the risk of fracture is reduced by 50% following 5 years' HRT, although the benefit reduces with cessation of treatment. It is safe to administer HRT for 5 years and there are few contraindications. There is a small increased risk of breast cancer if HRT is given for more than 5 years. HRT will reduce bone loss if it is started at any age following the menopause.

Whom to treat?

All postmenopausal women are at risk, but those with low bone mass or known risk factors are at most risk (see pages 37–8). The attitudes of doctor and patient exclude far more patients than do true contraindications.

Whom not?

Absolute contraindications:

- Breast carcinoma
- Endometrial carcinoma
- Undiagnosed uterine bleeding ⎫
- Pregnancy   ⎬ should be resolved first
- Uncontrolled hypertension   ⎭
- Severe present thromboembolic disease
- Severe liver disease.

Relative contraindications

There is little evidence to support the following group of contraindications. They are seldom a reason for a woman not to take HRT if it is indicated. Remember that natural doses are being used of hormones to which the woman has been exposed naturally for many years concurrent with these 'risks'. Assessment of the risk of osteoporosis should be weighed against the risk from these conditions.

Common conditions:

- Myocardial infarct
- Cerebrovascular accident
- Hypertension
- Thromboembolic disease
- Abnormal lipid profile
- Breast dysplasia
- Uterine fibroids
- Obesity
- Heavy smoking
- Cholelithiasis.

Uncommon conditions:

- Active or oestrogen-related liver disease
- Malignant melanoma
- Endometriosis
- Family history of breast carcinoma before 40 years
- Renal disease
- Severe diabetes
- Familial hyperlipidaemia.

When to treat?

Treatment is most effective if it is started as soon as possible after the menopause, as bone mass, once lost, cannot be restored to normal. It is probably of no advantage to start before menstruation ceases, and it becomes uncertain whether the woman is still fertile.

There is some benefit at all higher ages as the rate of bone loss is reduced.

How long?

HRT for 5 years reduces the risk of fracture by 50%, but hormone-related bone loss is prevented for as long as HRT is continued. This benefit is gradually lost on stopping HRT.

The risk of breast cancer is not significantly increased with 5 years' treatment, but is increased with longer treatment and the risk/benefit ratio has to be reassessed and the patient counselled if treatment for more than 5 years is considered.

What benefits are there?

The risk of fracture is reduced by 50%. The risks of ischaemic heart disease and of stroke are reduced with oestrogens.

What risks?

The risk of carcinoma of the uterus is increased with unopposed oestrogens, but not with combined oestrogen/progestogen therapy.

The risk of carcinoma of the breast is increased by more than 5 years' treatment and increases with duration of treatment.

The risk of venous thromboembolic events is slightly increased.

What screening at initiation?

The patient must be counselled about the menopause, osteoporosis and HRT.

A physical examination should include:

- Weight
- Blood pressure
- A pelvic examination
- A cervical smear (if this has not been carried out in the previous 3 years)

- A breast examination
- Mammography (if it is available).

Gynaecological referral is recommended if there is irregular or postmenopausal bleeding before HRT is commenced.

No routine endometrial biopsy is necessary if combined oestrogen/progestogen therapy is used, and if there is amenorrhoea or a regular cycle.

What side-effects?

Bleeding is usual with cyclical combined HRT. The periods may be heavy, but they usually become lighter after a few months. Bleeding occurs in the first 6 months in up to 20% of women taking continuous combined HRT. Gynaecological referral is recommended if there are irregular or abnormal bleeds.

Breast tenderness is common, but usually settles after 2–3 months. Other side-effects are uncommon: they include increased nipple sensitivity, nausea and vomiting, fluid retention and depression.

Most side-effects resolve with continuing treatment, or after changing the dose of oestrogen or the type of progestogen.

Headaches are an important side-effect: stop HRT if migrainous or focal headaches start for the first time. Migraine or headaches before treatment are not a guide to the risk of headaches or migraine on HRT.

What advice to patients?

Patients should be given a clear explanation of the menopause and the risks and benefits of HRT. They should be warned that menstruation will probably return but not fertility (although some women are fertile in the early menopause). If HRT is commenced before the cessation of periods, they must be informed that it will not act as a contraceptive. One should discuss the common side-effects and the monitoring of treatment, and encourage compliance.

What monitoring?

There should be follow-up visits at 3 and 9 months, and then every 6–12 months. This should include assessment of:

- Symptom control
- Side-effects
- Bleeding pattern
- Blood pressure
- Weight.

The annual visit should also include:

- Breast examination (encourage self-examination)
- Pelvic examination.

Every 3 years there should be:

- Mammogram as part of standard screening programmes
- Cervical smear
- Endometrial biopsy if the patient is taking unopposed oestrogens. With combination oestrogen/progesterone an endometrial biopsy is only required if there is breakthrough bleeding.

When to stop?

The benefit is greater with continued use, but 5 years' treatment will confer a significant reduction in risk of future fracture. If the patient wishes to continue HRT for more than 5 years (many do), she should be counselled concerning the increased risk of carcinoma of the breast.

The appearance of serious side-effects, increased anxiety or the development of a contraindication are all reasons to stop HRT.

What responds best to hormone replacement therapy?

The disorders associated with the menopause can be divided into the autonomic, the psychogenic and the metabolic (Table 15).

Table 15 *Disorders of the menopause*

Autonomic	Psychogenic	Metabolic
Hot flushes	Insomnia	Osteoporosis
Sweats	Apprehension	Ischaemic heart disease
Palpitations	Headaches	Skin atrophy
Dizziness	Depression	Urge incontinence
Globus hystericus	Anxiety	Vaginal dryness, dyspareunia
Formication	Libido changes	
	Loss of concentration	

The response rates to HRT vary for these different problems (Table 16). The autonomic and psychogenic disorders respond early, if at all, to HRT, but the metabolic disorders, such as vaginal dryness and 'cystitis' (urethral irritation or urge incontinence), can take months and the prevention of cardiovascular disease and osteoporosis takes years.

Table 16 *Which menopausal symptoms respond best to hormone replacement therapy?*

% who benefit	Symptom
70–80	Hot flushes
60–70	Night sweats
50–60	Irritability
40–50	Depression Tiredness Ability to cope Nervous tension
30–40	Trouble sleeping Ability to concentrate
20–30	Headaches, crying spells, palpitations Aches and pains Feelings of panic Pain/difficulty with sex

With what if the uterus is intact?

In the first few years after the menopause combined HRT should be given, with continuous oestrogen to control menopausal symptoms and a progestogen for at least 12 days per cycle to convert a proliferative endometrium into its secretory phase prior to menstruation.

Most women will menstruate (but need reassurance that they cannot become pregnant – a real concern of some women – unless HRT was commenced before the menopause or in the early menopause).

Natural oestrogens (oestradiol, oestriol, or conjugated equine oestrogens) are preferred. The minimum effective doses to prevent osteoporosis are: 2 mg oestradiol; 0.625 mg conjugated equine oestrogens or a plasma oestradiol concentration of 150–200 μmol/l after percutaneous administration. Various combination hormone products are commercially available.

After 2 years from the menopause continuous combined oestrogen with progestogen, tibolone or raloxifene can be considered.

With what in hysterectomized women?

Continuous oestrogens should be given. There is no benefit in mimicking the natural cycle with an oestrogen/progestogen combination. As for women with the uterus intact, natural oestrogens are preferred and the minimum dose is the same.

SERMs

Raloxifene is a selective oestrogen receptor modulator (SERM) that is indicated for the prevention and treatment of osteoporosis. It has been shown to improve bone mass in hip and spine and to reduce the risk of vertebral fractures. It is an agonist for oestrogen receptors in bone, but an antagonist for receptors in the uterus and breast. There is no vaginal bleeding and the risk of breast cancer is reduced. There are favourable effects on biochemical markers of cardiovascular risk. There is an increased risk of venous thromboembolism and some women have hot flushes, especially if it is started close to the menopause.

Calcium

Calcium ions are essential for the function of all living cells. Ionized calcium in the blood is precisely regulated by hormones and the bones act as a reservoir (of total body calcium, 99% is in the bones). The absorption of dietary calcium is incomplete (Figure 25).

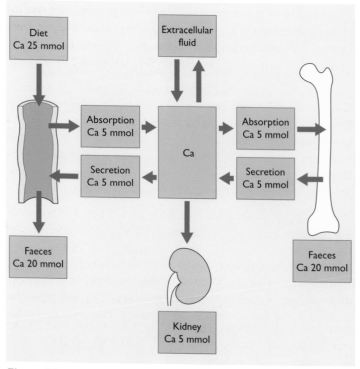

Figure 25 *Daily calcium turnover.*

Regulation of calcium metabolism

The extracellular calcium concentration is precisely controlled, largely by three hormones: parathyroid hormone, vitamin D and calcitonin.

Parathyroid hormone (PTH) maintains plasma calcium. Its secretion by the parathyroid glands is stimulated by a fall in plasma calcium. It increases renal tubular reabsorption of calcium, increases intestinal calcium absorption by stimulating renal synthesis of 1,25-vitamin D, and increases bone resorption.

Vitamin D is necessary for the normal mineralization of bone, and deficiency results in osteomalacia; it also promotes intestinal calcium absorption. Vitamin D occurs in fish oils and some dairy foods, but the most important source is the skin by the action of UV light on 7-dehydrocholesterol. The potent metabolites 25-hydroxy-vitamin D and 1,25-dihydroxy-vitamin D are then formed by hydroxylation in liver and kidney, respectively. Synthesis of 1,25-dihydroxy-vitamin D is stimulated by parathyroid hormone.

Calcitonin decreases bone resorption. It is synthesized by the C cells of the thyroid gland. Secretion is stimulated by an increase in plasma calcium.

Calcium and bones

An adequate calcium intake is important at all stages of life.

Epidemiological studies show a positive correlation between long-term calcium intake and bone mass, with a reduced frequency of hip fracture. Attainment of peak bone mass is impaired by persistently low calcium intakes. Calcium absorption declines with age, although the exact mechanism for this is unclear, and a normal dietary calcium intake is insufficient to maintain calcium balance.

Bone loss at the menopause is not significantly influenced by calcium intake, but dietary calcium of 1000 mg daily is recommended to maintain calcium balance.

Table 17 *Recommended daily dietary allowances for calcium (adapted from* Report on Osteoporosis in the European Community: Action for prevention. *Luxembourg, European Communities, 1998.)*

Group	Age (years)	Range (mg)
Newborn	0–0.5	400
Children	1–3	400–600
	4–6	450–600
	7–10	550–700
Men	11–24	900–1000
	25–65	700–800
	65–	700–800
Women	11–24	900–1000
	25–50	700–800
	50–65	800
	65–	700–800
Pregnant		700–900
Lactating		1200

Calcium in large doses (1000–1500 mg daily) in postmenopausal women and in established osteoporosis reduces the rate of bone loss – of cortical bone, in particular – although it is not as effective as HRT. It inhibits remodelling and osteoclastic bone resorption. It is most effective in those who have a low calcium intake. Calcium can be taken in the diet or as supplements, which are well tolerated and inexpensive.

The recommended daily dietary allowances of calcium are given in Table 17.

The dietary sources of calcium are dairy products (1 pint milk, skimmed or whole, contains 700 mg; 1 oz Cheddar cheese 200 mg; 5 oz yoghurt 250 mg), tinned fish, green vegetables and dietary supplements.

Calcium and vitamin D

Calcium 1.2 g/day with vitamin D 800 IU is effective at preventing non-vertebral fractures in the frail elderly, who are probably relatively deficient in both.

Vitamin D and calcitriol

Vitamin D supplements in high doses appear to be of no value. Activated vitamin D – calcitriol – probably reduces the risk of vertebral and non-vertebral fractures and can be used to treat osteoporosis.

Bisphosphonates

Bisphosphonates reduce bone resorption by inhibiting the activity of osteoclasts. Three bisphosphonates – etidronate, alendronate and risedronate – are widely available for the treatment of osteoporosis. They are also effective in steroid-induced osteoporosis. Bisphosphonates are used to treat Paget's disease and hypercalcaemia.

Bisphosphonates bind to calcium in food, which inhibits their absorption. They must be taken on an empty stomach with tap water. Even mineral water will reduce absorption.

The optimum duration of treatment is not yet established. The benefit is seen within the first year, but treatment is usually considered to be long term.

Cyclical etidronate increases bone mass and reduces the risk of vertebral fractures. Observational studies also suggest protection from hip fractures. The suggested regimen is etidronate 400 mg daily for 14 days followed by calcium 500 mg daily for 76 days, repeating the cycle over several years. It is well tolerated.

Alendronate also increases bone mass and has been shown in randomized controlled trials to reduce the risk of vertebral and non-vertebral fractures. For prevention 5 mg/day and for treatment 10 mg/day or 70 mg/week are recommended. A small risk of oesophagitis has become apparent in clinical use, but was not found in studies. To minimize this risk alendronate is taken first thing in the morning with a tumbler of water, the patient remaining upright and taking no food or tablets for at least 30 minutes.

Risedronate has recently become available. It increases bone mass and has been shown in randomized controlled trials to reduce the risk of vertebral and non-vertebral fractures. It was well tolerated in studies. The recommended dose for prevention and treatment of osteoporosis is 5 mg/day. It is also recommended to be taken first thing in the morning with a tumbler of water, the patient remaining upright and taking no food or tablets for at least 30 minutes

Other bisphosphonates, including **ibandronate** and **zoledronate**, are still under investigation.

Calcitonin

Calcitonin reduces bone resorption and the rate of bone loss. It is available by injection and as an intranasal spray. Trials have used the different preparations and show a reduction in the risk of vertebral and non-vertebral fractures, although the benefits may be fewer than those found with bisphosphonates.

There is some analgesic effect and calcitonin is of use for an acute vertebral fracture, although the mechanism of this effect is unclear. The suggested dose for this effect is 100 IU by injection daily for 21 days. The commonest side-effect is flushing.

Calcitonin is administered by injection or intranasal spray: the dose suggested to reduce bone loss varies from 50 IU three times weekly to 100 IU by injection daily or 200 IU intranasally. Treatment is currently recommended for 3 years.

Parathyroid hormone

Parathyroid hormone (PTH) maintains extracellular calcium levels and has anabolic properties on bone. Trials of recombinant PTH have shown a reduction in the risk of vertebral and non-vertebral fractures with a dose-dependent increase in bone density. When available, it will open up treatment options for severe cases of osteoporosis.

Male osteoporosis

Testosterone may reduce the rate of bone loss in established male osteoporosis and should be considered if hypogonadism is demonstrated. In view of the uncertain benefit at present, specialist supervision with facilities to monitor bone density is advised.

Bisphosphonates are also effective in men.

Exercise

Physical activity affects bone mass, trabecular architecture and bone remodelling; immobilization results in rapid bone loss. Physical activity at all ages increases bone mass. Furthermore, exercise improves general fitness, coordination, strength and reaction time and reduces the risk of a traumatic fall.

Weight-bearing exercises are the most effective for maintaining bone mass, and 3 hours of aerobic exercises per week has been shown to reduce bone loss in menopausal women.

Excessive exercise in young women can cause amenorrhoea, and bone mass is reduced compared to that of eumenorrhoeic colleagues. That is to say, oestrogen is more important than exercise. It is best to recommend a daily programme of warm-up exercises, general exercises to include jogging and dance-oriented exercises, and hard walking to total at least 1 hour per day.

Hip protectors

The impact of falls can be reduced by external hip protectors, and these should be considered in frail elderly with a history of falls.

Preventing falls

A fracture will usually have followed a trauma – typically a fall – and fallers are at risk of further falls. Risk factors for falling should be identified and, where possible, corrected (see page 34).

Appendix:
Common questions
and concerns

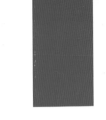

Is it hereditary?

There is an increased risk of osteoporosis if there is a strong family history, but this is only one of many risk factors. It is not a good predictor of who will or will not fracture. Patients can be reassured, but on the other hand they know from experience what osteoporosis is and are often the most enthusiastic patients for preventive therapy with HRT and the most likely to take it long term.

Can I get pregnant while on HRT, as I am having periods?

A common question. In rare cases in the early menopause, or if HRT is started before the menopause, women might be fertile as there would be insufficient hormones to suppress ovulation.

Does HRT cause cancer?

A real concern and the commonest reason why women do not want to take HRT. There is no significant increased risk of uterine cancer with combination HRT, and no significant increased risk of breast cancer with HRT for 5 years.

Can I take HRT, as I didn't get on with the pill?

HRT uses low natural doses of oestrogen and progestogen. It may cause problems that the patient had with the normal menstrual cycle, but not with the contraceptive pill.

What diet should I take?

The only important thing about diet is adequate calcium intake (see pages 72–4). Excessive amounts of protein or bran may impair calcium balance.

What exercise should I do?

All exercise is good. Weight-bearing exercises are best for the skeleton (see pages 53–62).

Should I wear a corset?

Corsets seldom help. The thoracic spine is usually affected and cannot be supported by a corset. The abdomen protrudes because of the loss of height, and a corset worsens the feeling of fullness, reflux oesophagitis and stress incontinence.

What symptoms are attributable to osteoporosis?

Osteoporosis only causes symptoms if there has been a fracture. It does not cause generalized skeletal pain or generalized back pain without evidence of fracture. Height loss can be due to disc degeneration, and a radiograph is necessary to distinguish between the two (see pages 46–7).

Is it too late to treat a patient who has osteopenia?

Is it too late to treat a patient who has sustained a hip fracture?

It is never too late to treat any patient, and a reduction in the risk of fracture is seen after a year of use of some treatments. It is as important to prevent the elderly from falling.

This patient cannot take HRT because she had a deep vein thrombosis (DVT) on the contraceptive pill/during pregnancy

Most women who have had a DVT will have continued to expose themselves naturally to cyclical oestrogen and progestogen for many years without a recurrence. There is no reason why HRT, using 'natural' doses, should suddenly precipitate a recurrent DVT.

The treatment for my osteoporosis has not helped my back pain

Treatments to reduce further bone loss, such as HRT or calcium, do not relieve pain, although calcitonin may do so.

When should I refer to hospital?

The risk of future osteoporosis is at present best assessed by bone-mass measurement after midlife. This is available in specialist centres.

Further information

International Osteoporosis Foundation (IOF)
71, cours Albert-Thomas
69447 Lyon Cedex 03
France

www.osteofound.org

For patients in the UK, further information is available from:

National Osteoporosis Society (NOS)
Camerton
Bath BA2 0PJ

Tel: 01761 471771 (for general enquiries)
Tel: 01761 472721 (for medical queries)
Fax: 01761 471104

e-mail: info@nos.org.uk
www.nos.org.uk

Index

Page numbers in *italics* indicate figures or tables.